Rapid Weight Loss Hypnosis For Women: Beginners Guided Meditations & Self-Hypnosis For Burning Fat, Overcoming Food Addiction, Eating Healthy Including Positive Affirmations

By Meditation Made Effortless

Table of Contents

"…" means take a breath while speaking before you continue.

PAUSE (for a few breaths)

LONGER PAUSE (give time to allow the listener time to imagine what you've suggested)

Introduction

Thank you for picking up the Rapid Weight Loss for women hypnosis audio... this surely is a sign of self-love and it only means that you want to burn fat and slim down...to be able to feel and look great. And...hypnosis can get you started on this effortless weight loss journey.

Pause

So, congratulations for taking this step towards a fitter and happier YOU...please listen to this audio using headphones... so that the sound of my voice is clear and if you lose track of me and your mind starts to wander...you can easily tune back into the sound of my voice.

Pause

Do not listen to this audio...when your mind needs you to be conscious such as while operating machinery or driving. Listen to this audio... when you are in a comfortable position...sitting on a chair or resting on a bed.

Pause

One last note, hypnotherapists usually work with their patients for 6-12 sessions to achieve lasting results with Weight Loss hypnotherapy, therefore, we recommend you go through these Hypnosis around 6-12 times over the next couple of weeks/ months, ideally commit to several chapters of this book each day.

However, each situation is unique and can depend on you, your mental state and the intensity of change you want to being into your life. Therefore, while we offer 6-12 sessions as a recommendation, this is not set in stone and you may need more or less. After each set of sessions, see how you feel, and then decide if you need more.

We also recommend sticking to one set of recordings over a period of time, rater than chopping and changing. For example, you may also have our Sleep Hypnosis, but we recommend completing this one, fully first before moving on to that one.

Now, sit back and relax, it's time to get started.

Let us start... 5 Minutes

Begin recording

Induction

You are now listening to the sound of my voice... and the sound of my voice only ...and as you continue to listen to each word I say...you allow yourself to relax more and more.

Pause

I wonder if you could take a deep breath...hold it for a count of 5... and then exhale.

Pause

Let's start now.

Breathe in Deeply...

Pause

Hold for a count of 5

1... 2...3...4...and 5

Now, exhale...

Pause

Once more, take another deep breath...

Breathe in...

Hold for a count of 5 — 1, 2, 3, 4, 5 (slowly)

Now, breathe out...

Pause

Once more, take another deep breath —

Breathe in

Hold for a count of 5 — 1, 2, 3, 4, 5 (slowly)

Now, breathe out

Pause

And, come back to your normal breathing pattern...

Pause

— And, I wonder… if you could simply bring all your focus and attention to the center of your eye-brows…with your eyes closed…try to look at the center of your brows and focus on the point between them…that's right.

Pause

In a moment, I am going to talk to that part of you, which is highly creative…the part that knows exactly how to help you imagine or create anything with the help of your mind's eye.

Pause

And… I know you can do it… because everybody can…we all have a creative mind, that has the ability and capability to create and imagine images in our mind.

I know you must have imagined or visualized or day-dreamed many times in your life.

And... our creative part helps us imagine and visualize. Isn't it?

With the help of our creative mind, we can visualize, imagine, write, paint, and dream...and I am going to be talking to that part of you today.

Pause

Deepener

And, I wonder if that part of you can help you imagine… that you are laying on a beautiful grass, the grass is moist, and you can feel the wonderful moist grass beneath your feet…

Longer Pause (8 seconds pause)

The day is beautiful, the Sun is shining bright… and you can feel the warm sunshine touch your skin gently…

Pause

As you look around, you notice there are bushes and trees around you… and perhaps a stream of water somewhere nearby as you hear the magical sound of the water flowing…

Pause

There's a beautiful fragrance of flowers around you...and you can smell the fragrance of your favorite flowers... as you continue to imagine that, I wonder if you can notice a tree next to you. A tall tree...with many branches and green leaves having different shades of green...And, as you notice the trunk of the tree, you notice a black ant moving down the trunk to reach its roots visible just above the ground.

The tree seems quite old and strong...

You focus on it... and with every little distance it covers down the trunk...you find yourself drifting more and more and falling deeper and deeper into a beautiful state of relaxation...

Pause

Starting now...

10... Look at the movement of the ant

9 ...see how it moves down the tree trunk

8 ... drifting down and down

7 ... as it gets closer and closer to the ground

6 ... you start to feel even more relaxed

5 ... continuing to look at the ant's movement

4 ... feeling the relaxation in every part of your body

3 ... the ant is about to reach the tree roots

2 ...you are getting even more relaxed

1 ... the ant has reached the ground

0 ...You are now comfortably relaxed

Pause

You are now deeply and beautifully relaxed...

And as you focus on the sound of my voice...your imagination opens up even more...

And you notice a long corridor in front of you, with a door at the end of it.

Pause

Just imagine that you are in a long corridor or hallway...and as you notice that...you also notice its walls and the floor...and as you continue to notice that...you allow yourself to relax even more and you move forward towards the door...

Pause

And the door leads you...to a point on the road, where you make a decision about your life. The life that is full of confidence, high self-worth, hope, and positivity or the life that makes you insecure, frustrated, underconfident, and sad. You have a choice to make...an important decision to make. You are at the fork...at a decision point...

One road shows you the life where you see yourself as slim, attractive and confident...whereas the other road shows you the life where you continue to live the life you are already living...perhaps a life with no or less exercise and unhealthy eating.

The road that shows you as slim, confident, and attractive person, living a successful and happy life...is on the right whereas the left road... seems bumpy, dingy, and definitely not happy. Perhaps it's a road of misery...where you see yourself as just the way you are...continuing to live the life you are already living...

And, I wonder if you can take the road to the left and notice what all you see and how you feel.

Pause

Look at your body...your eating habits... your lifestyle...your relationships, do you feel happy seeing yourself on road left?

Pause

And, I wonder if you could see yourself on the same road five years from now… do you see yourself as pleased with yourself? Do you feel healthier or worse?

Get the knowing of it…

Pause

The time has come for you to come back to the fork and the point where you now need to go on the right path of happiness, health, and confidence…and then make a decision…the wise decision…the right decision. And, I know you can do it, because everybody can…

I wonder if you can take that road and see how your life looks like six months from now…the right road shows the active lifestyle…the healthy eating habits… the life where you have taken charge of your life… and emotions… and someone who is determined and focused to achieve daily goals... to achieve the big goal of slimming down and losing weight...isn't it?

Pause

And, I wonder if you could now look at yourself five years from now...living an active lifestyle and I wonder if you could get the knowing of the feelings around that lifestyle...

Do you feel smart about living this kind of life?

Pause

And, now that you have seen both the lives, I wonder if you are ready to make the decision to choose the life that gives you maximum happiness, positivity, hope, confidence, and self-worth...

Pause

And as I count from 3 to 1, you will choose the path that is right for you. The right path that will turn you into a successful, happy, and confident person.

Starting now…

3, 2, and 1.

That's right.

Longer Pause

Confidence and Self Esteem Script

Continuing to go deeper and deeper with every word I say and with every breath you take...you are now getting mentally, physically, and emotionally relaxed and are more receptive to what I say...

Pause

You are now ready to make important changes to your life and to your body that will make you live a happier and fulfilling life.

Pause

And as you continue to listen to me, you become aware of the times you felt low on confidence, perhaps a time in childhood, teens, or from anytime of your life.

You will be able to bring up those memories in black and white....as if you they are like old photo negatives we used to have decades ago.

Pause

And with the power of your mind...you can easily bring up those memories as photo negatives... where someone made you feel low about yourself or perhaps the times where you felt underconfident. Get the knowing of that...

Longer Pause

Notice all those events in the form of old photo negatives coming out of your body... perhaps from different parts of your body ...and moving towards the top of your head.

And as that happens, you feel your body getting lighter and lighter...

You know that they do not belong to you anymore and the today is the day to discard these from your system, your body, your thoughts, your emotions...that's right.

Pause

I don't know if you know that lack of confidence and low self-esteem generally originate from the childhood...perhaps coming from the situations involving teachers...critical parents, peers, friends that make you feel in a certain negative way about yourself.

This happens with most of us but the wise part of us know exactly what to do to be able to let go of these memories to live a better future...and not stay stuck in the past...

And...that part of you is now working for your highest good...

And as I talk to you...the subconscious is now going to make you imagine a bunch of helium balloons coming down from the sky...

Imagine a bunch of helium balloons is coming down to take away those images back to the sky, millions and millions of miles away....

I am going to count from 3 down to 1..and with each count down...the bunch is going to get bigger and bigger as it is going to come closer and closer...to take away that holds no value in your present...

3....2....1

Pause

And I wonder if you could now give away all those black and white photo negatives to the balloons and see them inside the balloons....

Notice how they look inside each balloon...

And, you can barely make out the memories as they look all blurred inside the balloons.

Pause

The time has come to let go of them...and feel liberated...absolutely free...and light...and when the balloons start to take a flight...you will feel free...as if the weight has been lifted...the old baggage...the unwanted...the not needed...that's right...it's all going to go now....away...far away... that's right.

In a moment, you will notice that the bunch of balloons takes a flight back to the universe...back to where it came from.... taking away all that does not solve any purpose.

You are now free from the feelings of low confidence and low self-esteem….as these are the things of past. You had experienced these emotions long time ago and you no longer give them importance as they hold no more importance.

You are free and feeling light mentally, emotionally, and physically.

That's right.

And, I wonder if you could now imagine a color of confidence. The color that resonates with confidence…imagine any color and the moment you imagine that color, you feel confident….

Pause

I wonder if you could now Imagine that color moving into your body and encompassing you from all sides.

As if you are inside the cocoon of confidence, exuding confidence from every part of your body.

And, this confidence helps you to be positive…energetic…happy… and joyful.

With confidence you can achieve all your health goals. That's right…especially the weight you want to be at, it's so much easier now to achieve it. Because you are confident. Absolutely confident about what you want to achieve and who you want to be soon.

You are now confident and this confidence is going to make losing weight easier and simpler. As you start to realise the fact that eating right…and exercising is the way to lose weight. It is 70 percent diet and 30 percent exercise…and if you follow this, you shall start to see the results in no time…

You lose weight when you eat right and exercise to burn off extra calories. This confidence helps you gain control on your eating habits and how you live your life...

If you know what to do, it gets easier to know how to do it... And, I know that you want to lose weight and you will figure out ways how to do that. Isn't it?

With high level of confidence, it gets easier for you to know the ways to achieve your goal weight. And, with every passing day, your self-esteem and self-worth is increasing....

And with every pound you lose, the confidence doubles up and you start to stay even more focused on your goals and this brings the feelings of self-respect...and self-worth. You feel energetic and has the profound sense of well-being.

You are well aware of your self-confidence inside of you you are self reliant, independent, and absolutely confident. You are full of determination, independence and you think confidently when making decisions. You are secure and you are ready to transform yourself fully from inside and outside.

You think and talk confidently...and its visible in your body language...you exude self confidence in your walk and how you behave with people...your friends and family are amazed to see you talk so confidently...

Pause

With this you are creating a positive reality for yourself having immense confidence self worth.self esteem positivity and happiness the inner joy that comes from assertiveness and the ability to make wise decisions for yourself..

Pause

Because of your positive attitude, positive thinking...and positive way of living...you experience a whole new reality in every area of your life whether its your work, relationships or health...

With every passing day you are getting stronger and stronger in your mind more assertive happier even more confident that's right...

Pause

You allow yourself to release all the fears and other negative emotions...that serve no purpose...and allow yourself to feel the positive emotions like security, freedom, positivity, happiness, confidence, calmness...contentment...

You are aligned and centred at all times... always looking at living your present day and living it mindfully to achieve the daily goals...living each day beautifully and productively.

You maintain calm and relaxed...focused and mindful. You are confident and secure about everything.

Pause

You are now receptive to all the suggestions for your highest good...to help you achieve your goal weight...

I would like you to now repeat the following affirmations after me in your mind.

I am confident and strong... (5 to 6 second pause)

I have high self esteem... (")

I am secure with myself... (")

I believe in myself ...(")

I am happy and joyous... (")

I take charge of my life...(")

I love myself...(")

I am happiness... (")

I am worthy of love...(")

I attract good things in life...(")

I have unique abilities...(")

I deserve success...(")

I deserve to be fit and healthy...(")

I respect myself...(")

I appreciate myself…(")

People appreciate me…(")

I am wonderful in everyway…(")

I am getting better with every passing day…(")

I deserve to be happy… (")

I am active, energetic, and positive…(")

Boost Your Metabolism

Your body is an expression of who you are inside...who you see yourself as. It shows your discipline and dedication in taking care of yourself. It also influences your sex appeal to others.

Before we start to work on your body, metabolism, exercising, and self-love, I wonder if you know that your outside is the reflection of your inside...to be able to slim down and burn fat, the work needs to be done inside for it to be reflected on the outside.

It is a mix of self-love...eating right...exercise...and proper sleep. And, before you even start taking actions to achieve what you want to achieve...you need to think first. So, I wonder if you can think about all the benefits you will have when achieve your ideal goal weight...

Longer Pause

And all change happens first in the mind... and listening to me only means you are broadening and widening your mind to receive positive information and let that information get absorbed so much so that it is reflected in your actions... Isn't it?

Because what you think, becomes your reality...

And if you think your body to be burning fat with high metabolism, then you will certainly make it your reality...as you see your body into the perfect body sooner than you realise...

To be able to do that I wonder if you can image your perfect body now...that's right... Imagine yourself brimming with vitality and health, just how you want your body and health to be.

Pause

And stay focused on this goal and bring all your focus and attention to this image of yours…. and as you do that, feel the healthy energy starting to get into you and this makes you even calmer and relaxed…

Pause

And imagine yourself at your goal weight… wearing the clothes that are looking great on you…picture yourself looking great.

Pause

Look at your face, your arms, chest, stomach, and legs. Observe every part of your body and once again imagine all the benefits of being at this goal weight.

Longer Pause (10 seconds pause)

You now have a goal in front of you… and you can only accomplish goals… if you have them. And, when you have a goal…you only need to take actions to reach the goals. Isn't it?

And achieving goals is easy and effortless…because you know the benefits of achieving goals and how you can feel, once you have achieved them.

And I wonder if you could feel what you will feel if you achieve the goal of attaining the ideal goal weight. How would you feel?

PAUSE

Stay with the feeling…

And, as you continue to listen to each word I say, you are feeling motivated to be successful at whatever you do.

Eating smaller portions

Exercise and proper diet increase the metabolism... and to be able to do that, you exercise at least 30 minutes every day and eat smaller portions 5- 6 times a day. When you eat frequent smaller portions...you are able to digest better, which in turns boosts the metabolism.

It also helps in stabilizing blood sugar levels and offer nutrients to the body the entire day...

To keep your metabolic rate high...feel less hungry...and have high levels energy, smaller portions of food is the key.

Increase metabolism by eating several smaller meals per day. The idea is to never let yourself get hungry...

And to achieve high metabolism...eat six smaller meals throughout the day instead of having three big meals. Divide your one big meal into two and have it in the gap of two to three hours. It is easy and this way you will never starve yourself...and save yourself from binge eating.

Pause

The way you will accomplish this is to eat healthy nutritious meals and
eat healthy nutritious snacks in between those meals keeping yourself satisfied
throughout the day. Include fruits and more salads in the diet to eat healthy and keep the stomach full with smaller portions.

And with this, you can notice that all body parts and organs are functioning at the optimal level... with a thought to improve the body through nutritious diet and exercising.

With every passing day...you can notice increase in your energy levels and the metabolism is becoming aligned with your needs.

You consciously and subconsciously reduce the portion size...to be able to eat the right amount of nutritious food...and you eat foods that are good for your health.

And this makes you feel so much relaxed and calm... as you continue to listen to each word I say.

Your metabolism gets adjusted when your body is at rest...you feel a sense of peace and calm within you and because of all the improvements taking place in your mind, your are able to pump more oxygen in your lungs and your heartbeat becomes steadier and breathing becomes natural.

This only means that your nervous system is beginning to function more appropriately...and all the organs are working harmoniously inside your body. That's right.

You are a confident person and believe in yourself...You can effortlessly and easily release all the extra weight to reach your ideal goal weight.

Pause

You are a lovable and confident person...you will eat only when you are hungry and not eat foods to pass time or eat when there is some emotional trigger... You will no longer food to give you the comforting feeling... because that only means you give all the power to the food and then the extra or junk food makes you be what you do not want to be.

So... you take charge of your life and take charge of your body.

And the more you do it... the better control you have on your eating and exercise habits. You notice that with every passing day... you are becoming focused on your goal and you take actions accordingly to accomplish it.

Pause

And now I wonder if you could imagine yourself as an attractive woman and as you begin to act and walk like a healthy and attractive woman, you manifest it...and make it your reality.

With paying attention to the portions and thoughts before taking extra food...you allow yourself to eat less and feel confident.

Pause

Imagine just deciding on eating smaller portions can already make you feel good about yourself...isn't it?

Through this recording, you are able to bring satisfaction which leads to relaxation and brings you a healthy, attractive, and slimmer body....

Get Rid of the Sweet Tooth

And you focus on the sound of my voice and allow yourself to go even deeper with every breath you take…and with every word I say.

And all these words sink into your subconscious mind effortlessly and you begin to feel even more comfy and relaxed….

If your food habits also include having desserts, sweetened drinks, and other sugary stuff then you may have difficulty in losing weight faster.

Pause

And you are listening to me because you want to get rid of the sweet tooth you have and end the sugar cravings forever. Isn't it?

Pause

And, I wonder if you can look into your mouth with your mind's eye for that tooth that makes you crave sweets and you know because of that you may not lose weight easily.

Longer Pause

And you have found it….and the time has come to talk to the tooth and understand the purpose of it…

Perhaps the purpose of the tooth is to eat sugars…and you know there are natural sugars in fruits that can satiate the tooth…without affecting your body.

Because you love yourself and are excited to meet your weight loss goals and be at your ideal goal weight…you are going to make a contract with the sweet tooth that it will only be happy with the sugars coming from fresh fruits and vegetables. You can substitute white sugar with raw honey or jaggery...that will make the tooth and you happy.

This will be a win - win situation for you both...and I know you can convince the sweet tooth...can't you?

Pause

You know that sugary fruits and artificially sweetened drinks and foods will convert the sugar into fat...that will harden the arteries, adding fat to the body, and also rotting the teeth.

Sweet Tooth is a part of your body and it is a small part of you...you cannot make it so big in your system...that it controls your eating habits and make you gain weight...isn't it?

You will turn the sweet tooth into a healthy tooth that is happy having natural sugars and you will be aware of all the foods having natural sugars, so that you only have those...and satiate the desire of the healthy tooth.

And the healthy tooth only craves healthy foods, natural sugars, lots of water, fruits and vegetables, and whole grains.

Pause

I wonder if you could go back to the time when you first loved having sugary foods...perhaps a time when you were much younger...

Longer Pause

And the adult part of you that is listening to this audio, has the capability to go to that time when the younger self of yours started loving sweets, perhaps chocolates, candies, and similar foods. Maybe your parents gave them to you to pacify you...

The time has come to meet the younger self and talk to the child about the long term bad effects of having too much sweet and sugary stuff...

And also tell the child about the benefits of having natural sugars...the effects it has on skin, gut, and overall mood.

I would like you to speak to the child as if it were your own...and talk to the child...

Longer Pause

And, once you have spoken to the child...take the child from that time back to this time....as I count from 3 to 1.

3, 2, and 1...

And, you are now back with the child...and the child knows all the benefits of having natural sugars and all the disadvantages of having artificial sweetened foods or foods loaded with sugar.

In a moment, you both will become one with each other as one individual who does not crave sugar anymore...and only loves to have natural sugars...

Imagine yourself now integrating into each other...make the child reside in your heart...and see yourself as one person who is excited to stick to the weight loss plan to reach the weight loss goal.

Longer Pause

You know sweet drinks and sweetened foods with sugar are like poison to your body.

And with this awareness, you are able to spot sugary foods easily and stop yourself from eating and drinking them...instead you think wisely and choose foods with natural sugars to satiate the craving and make yourself and the healthy tooth happy and satiated.

Pause

You are now one...someone who looks for sugar only in fruits...and you enjoy having fruits and vegetables.

And, now imagine yourself at the ideal goal weight...looking absolutely stunning...and attractive.

You know you have reached this goal only by making changes to your diet and including a regular exercise regimen in your routine....

How does it feel to be this successful?

Pause

LOW CARB DIET

And, I wonder… if you could now join me in a fun exercise where you will imagine a platter full of delicious and colourful fruits and vegetables.

Pause

As you take a look at the platter… you start to salivate as they look so fresh. They are farm fresh, tender…delicious and vibrant. Take a closer look at the fruits and vegetables…look at the skin of fruits and veggies, touch and smell them. Perhaps there is a bright green broccoli that is rich in protein and the vibrant carrot, full of vitamins…

Pause

You pick up what you really like and get attracted to, and bite into the deliciousness and freshness. And, as you do that... you feel the taste buds dancing with joy...

Longer Pause

You overlooked all these foods and their goodness from coming into your body before and today is the day to realise the value of these foods... You just made a decision to switch to a low-carb diet...another great and wise decision to live a healthy and active life.

Pause

You eat healthy foods to not only be healthy and to lose weight but also to be mentally alert. Healthy foods make you get through the day effortlessly and with lean proteins, fruits, veggies, and whole grains...you get minerals, vitamins and nutrients to keep yourself in optimal health....

Because it is important to balance carbohydrates and proteins, you take whole grains and lean proteins that are excellent source of energy...Vegetables, fruits, and whole grains have fibre in them that keeps you full for longer... The darker the veggies the more nutrients they have....

And you think of having a beautiful and glowy skin with the kind of body you desire...it is going to be a complete transformation...and you are so looking forward to living a life full of confidence, high self-esteem, active and slim body, and clear skin...and all this is possible with the wise decisions you have already made today...

Longer Pause

By making your first steps into the world of healthy foods...you experienced the joy of eating mindfully...of taking care of your diet as well as your body...thus promoting a healthy mind and body. You feel fitter, lighter, slimmer and overall great. That's right.

And I wonder, if you could now imagine that these low carb foods are entering your stomach. And because they are low on carbohydrates....low levels of insulin are secreted and because of the low calorie or low carb diet...the body uses stored up fat for energy and leaves no room for fat backlog...which helps you to lose weight.

Pause

And with your great imagination, I wonder if you could, Imagine how clean your stomach looks from inside, take a closer look at the intestines, it's a happy stomach...isn't it?

And, with light and happy stomach, you feel so energised and full of vibrancy...

Pause

You now know the advantages of eating low calorie diet and some of the benefits are weight loss...fat reduction...high levels of energy...and livelier you.

And, I wonder if you can now tick off the low calorie and non- starchy, protein rich foods like lean meat, fish, beans, succulent fruits and vegetables...in your mind somewhere...

Pause

And that only means that ...from today on, you will be eating more of these foods to keep your stomach and yourself happy. Absolutely loving each smaller meal and moving towards your ideal goal weight.

Pause
You eat mindfully, embracing protein rich...low carb foods. Your diet includes

colourful fruits, vegetables. You consciously make efforts to reduce the portion size and increase the frequency of meals to six meals per day.

You drink at least eight glasses of water every day. Eating right is your new everyday goal to reach the bigger goal of release extra fat and weight to be able to reach your goal weight.

Pause

And I would like you to repeat the suggestions in your mind after me...

I eat healthy foods (4 seconds pauses)

I eat smaller portions (4 seconds pauses)

I exercise regularly (4 seconds pauses)

I am conscious of my eating habits (4 seconds pauses)

I eat mindfully (4 seconds pauses)

I exercise regularly (4 seconds pauses)

Pause

Be Motivated to Exercise

And you are now wondering how much exercise you are getting everyday and you know to be able to fasten the metabolism and lose weight easily, you need to also exercise in addition to eating right...

And I wonder if you could imagine a control room somewhere in your brain...perhaps it looks like a room with wires, knobs, buttons with lights flickering...

Longer Pause

You look at the control panel and you know to be able to control the functions in your mind and body, you need to fix something in here...

I don't know what that is ....but you know...

That's right..

Pause

You continue to look around in the control room and find a knob for exercise...and it has numbers around the knob from 0 to 10...perhaps the knob's indicator is set at a lower number and that causes you to procrastinate when it comes to exercising.

To be able to stay motivated and exercise every day...you may want to turn up the knob to a higher number...

Pause

And this only means that you will be excited every day to finish your workout session...because with every workout session you feel happier and confident about yourself...

This is one way to boost confidence and feel amazing…

And, perhaps there is a light flickering in the control room and that is the light of procrastination…and its flickering only means that its activated…and to be able to switch it off…you may want to cut the power cord….

You have the equipment to cut it now…

Cut now…that's right..

Pause

You have cut all cords with procrastination…because it never helped you…but only made you feel sad and guilty of not taking actions..

And, now you are free…liberated from the ties of procrastination…

Pause

You now start to wonder which exercise program will help you and you may begin to think that exercise is all about having a regimen that includes cardiovascular activity, some weight lifting, and stretching.

Pause

You begin to wonder that how many steps do you walk everyday...perhaps you need to walk a bit more and have a pedometer on your phone or some app to track the steps...

Pause

And you begin to feel active and energetic as soon as you finish walking 5000 steps a day. You add some more exercises to the routine...perhaps few Yoga Asanaas, pilates...or aerobics....and your mind choose the exercises that will bring maximum benefit to your body and help you achieve your weight goal really fast.

And with every passing day, you begin to realise that it's so much easier to exercise just like how you brush your teeth or take a shower and make exercise a part of your routine….effortless..

Pause

Sometimes you just stretch your legs and arms to feel relaxed and perhaps do some Pilates or aerobics by following an instructor on a video.

You can even just dance freestyle every day on your favorite dance numbers because the idea is to move your body and let the heart race to feel the burn and sweat to lose weight much faster…

And, I would like you to say the following suggestions in your mind after me..

I exercise everyday

(Pause for 5 seconds)

I move your body more

(Pause for 5 seconds)

I set exercise goals for every day

(Pause for 5 seconds)

I enjoy your exercise program

(Pause for 5 seconds)

I sweat and feel great

(Pause for 5 seconds)

I look forward to my exercise session every morning

Say No to Emotional Eating

And, as you continue to focus on the sound of my voice...I wonder if you could imagine a big projector screen in front of you....

Pause

And on the screen...you see yourself just before the time the emotional eating started. Perhaps it was few months ago or....a few years ago. I know you can easily access that memory, because everybody can.

Pause

Because a part of you can go through all the relevant memories that led you to start eating emotionally or when emotions overpowered you so much so, that you looked forward to eating food to feel happy and comfortable.

Pause

And, as that part of you looks for these memories... it can find the hidden emotion and you know many people with emotional eating issues discover that events led to emotional or comfort eating cause us to feel shame or guilt...and while looking for the events and emotions, you can easily begin...to notice how the series of events move backwards on the screen and then move forward like a fast forward.

Pause

That's right... you notice this happening quite a few times, until the events related to emotional eating get blurred and the images get totally distorted.

Longer Pause

And let the emotions related to those events simply get distorted with the images and you begin to form new coping strategies for success and achievement.

Pause

And as you continue to go deeper and deeper... listening to each word I say, I wonder if you know that the subconscious mind learns much faster than you can imagine....

Pause

And, that is why, you are now receptive to every positive word I say that will help you achieve a slimmer and fitter body...

I wonder if you could know the purpose of a refrigerator and the purpose is to keep the vegetables, fruits, milk, eggs, and much more fresh. And, similarly, the purpose of a vehicle is to take us to different places...isn't it?

Similarly, can you know the purpose of your feelings?

Pause

And, maybe you are struggling to know the purpose...

Sometimes, feelings of boredom's purpose is to make us overeat and the feelings of sadness's purpose is to again make us order in and eat junk food...

Sometimes, feelings of anxiety can cause us to overeat...and what action we take is a reaction to a feeling.

And overeating or eating junk food only makes us feel happy for a temporary moment and then causes us to feel guilty...and that's the beginning of a vicious cycle...

The feelings of guilt may again lead us to eat more... and then ultimately make us overweight...

Pause

So, eating in response to a feeling does not satisfy hunger...it only give a temporary relief and distracts us from a particular negative feeling.

And, as you continue to listen to what I say...you now know that you did not have any idea what needs to be done with the feelings. And, some people ignore them, some hide them, and some people distract themselves... by eating more.

And I wonder if you know that how the alarms goes off when you have to go for a meeting...indicating you to get up on time to reach office. If you do not pay attention to it, you may miss going to the meeting, which may have other consequences.

So similarly....alarm as an indicator asks you to take an action, but the action need to be the right action, which is to get up and start getting ready for the meeting....

And not take the action gets you in the loop of feeling the negative feelings again like frustration or guilt.

So, anytime a negative feeling arises, you need to think twice before taking an action. If you are feeling lonely, instead of picking up the phone to order food in, you may want to pick the phone to call your family or friends...

Pause

If you are feeling sad or stressed, instead of overeating... you may want to practice coping strategies like watching something funny... taking deep breaths, journaling the thoughts, or distracting your mind to do something else and feel a different feeling...

From now on, whenever you get a feeling and it's not hunger, you show yourself a red light- the stop light where you think twice and take the right action to not get into the loop of negative feelings. I know you can do it, because everybody can.

You are more aware of when you are actually physically hungry as compared to when you are hungry to satisfy emotions.

Pause

It gets easier for you to recognise feelings just before eating that is it the stomach that is hungry or the mind?

If it's the mind, then how can I distract my mind and take different actions to be able to divert myself from eating.

You may want to go for a walk or have a tall glass of water

Or talk to your family or play with your pet...

There are many ways to divert your mind to be able to take right actions and not eat in response of emotions.

Pause

And, when you are in control of your emotions, you get pleasure and satisfaction and you feel even more confident about yourself.

You are more ready than ever to feel happy, positive, fit, and confident...

And, with this feeling, you begin to realise that you can be calm, relaxed, and think wisely when it comes to taking actions.

Even when the challenges come, you are calm and relaxed and take actions when you have given much thought to it...

Your confidence continues to increase with every passing day, knowing you deserve to feel healthy and fit at your ideal goal weight.

Pause

You then use every other action that stops you from overeating or eating unhealthy foods.

And I want you to repeat the following suggestions in your mind after me...

I am conscious of my feelings

Pause

I am mindful of my actions

Pause

I love myself and think twice before taking actions

Pause

I am confident and believe in myself...

Heal Your Body

I wonder… if you could now imagine a beautiful and warm golden energy coming from the Sun. The beautiful Sun that gives the planet all the light and energy…

And imagine the energy or Sun light touching your head like a sharp beam …

The energy from the Sun is positive and healing and you can feel it moving into the top of your head…feel it inside of your head and perhaps with your third eye…see it moving into every cell and fibre of it.

That's right.

Imagine all the thoughts about past that no longer serve purpose and only make you feel negative in a certain way are moving out of your head… All those limiting beliefs about yourself... that you created or perhaps the labels given to you by others. All of those have no value in your life...and all those can't stop you from moving ahead in life.

Pause

As soon as the golden healing light touches every part of your mind, the beliefs about your body that you created at some point in life...the negative beliefs... those will simply go away.

Because the positive energy from the Sun clears your mind of all the negative thoughts and limiting beliefs that have no more value and serve no purpose...you allow yourself to let that happen...because this is the time to love yourself even more.

Pause

And it starts to further move down...towards your eyes...making you feel even more relaxed as you continue to listen to each word I say.

Further down to your facial muscles…cheeks, upper lips…jaws, and chin. Relaxing every part and muscle in your face…feeling the sense of calm in every part of your face.

And this happens, you begin to feel very comfortable in your own skin and start to love yourself more and more…

You now imagine the beautiful Sun's energy moving into your shoulders…taking away unwanted burdens that you may have.

Feel the energy into your shoulders, giving them all the comfort as you notice the energy moving into them with your mind's eye. Feel all the stress and burden taken away as the energy reaches your shoulders…

Pause

And, allow that beautiful golden energy, the comforting energy to touch your heart chakra, the center of your chest, and that's the seat of self-love. Imagine it moving down from your shoulders to the center of your chest...

Pause

And, I wonder if you could imagine activating the heart chakra and visualize the golden color turning green and moving in a clock-wise direction...Imagine this chakra moving like a fan or wheel in a clockwise direction...and this only means that you have started to love yourself even more. That's right.

Pause

And as you notice it moving like a fan or wheel ... you notice all the blockages in the heart chakra to be simply melting away. These blockages are stuck emotions related to past events or perhaps they are some worries. And, clearing the chakra and activating it with the green energy only means you are now activating the heart chakra to be able to bring self-love.

Longer Pause

The energy now moves into your arms, relaxing your arm muscles. Reaching every cell and fiber of your arms...making your arms and hands so very relaxed...that's right.

Pause

It now further moves down to your waist...and torso...and as this happens, you feel the sense of deep appreciation for yourself.

Pause

And as it continues to move down into your hips and thighs, you drift deeper and deeper into self-love. That's right.

And you can notice the golden light making its way into the wrists and fingers...

And as that happens, you tighten your fists and say to yourself. – "I can do it" That's right.

You can do it.

You can achieve all the goals that you have set for yourself on this weight loss journey...

Pause

The everyday goals to eat healthy to achieve the big goal of achieving your ideal weight. Isn't it?

You can see the energy moving into your feet and toes. Making you feel so relaxed, calm and at the same time positive and energetic...just like sun.

And you feel so determined to achieve the weight loss goals. I know you can do it because everybody can.

Pause

You now notice your whole body filled with golden healing energy...

This also has the power to melt the fat stored in your every part of your body…that perhaps make you look overweight or chubby…

Imagine all the fat getting melted…

you have the power to get rid of all the accumulated fat…

Longer Pause

And in a moment, you will notice that the light of self-love is melting the fat stored in your body. And with every breath you take and with every rise and fall of your chest, you can easily visualize fat melting away from your thighs, hips, stomach and other body part that has extra fat.

Longer Pause

You can do it

Pause

You know exactly how to lose weight

Pause

You are smart and very intelligent to make right decisions

Pause

You take actions every day to achieve daily goals

Pause

You love yourself even more with every passing day

Pause

You love your body

Pause

You are mindful and enjoy the present moment

Pause

You are slimming now

You are slimming Now

And, as you continue to relax even more… with every breath you take and with every word I say…it is even more easier for you feel and see what we are going to do…

My words are getting embedded in your mind… for your highest good…for you to achieve your weight loss goal. You have decided to not only lose weight but also tone and slim the body to look your best…

Pause

Because of the extra weight and fat, you may have experienced situations where you felt uncomfortable about your body, whether it was wearing a short dress or going into the pool. Because of the extra weight, you could not wear your favorite dresses and could not feel comfy in the clothes you were wearing. Isn't it?

Pause

And...you may have felt embarrassment, anger, frustration, shame, insecurity and sadness because of the extra weight you had been carrying.

Imagine if this continues to go on, how would you feel after a year or two years? Maybe sad again. Isn't it?

Longer Pause

You do not have to worry about living the same life after a year or two years because you are listening to me and you have already decided to change your body and change your life. Isn't it?

But now, there is no chance of going back to that life... living those negative emotions every day. You now know how important it is to lose weight and get slim.

Pause

You are ready to change... because slimming will transform every area of your life... Your health...your relationships...your work...and of course the most important area of self. You will have a beautiful relationship with yourself.

With new attitude, you have new hopes and positivity to take your life to the next level.

The moment you start to slim down and lose weight...you feel hopeful and positive and life seems so much better.

You are hopeful and it does not matter...how much you tried in the past, you know that this time, you are going to achieve your ideal goal weight. Every new action towards your goal will free you from your past and in no time, you will see the results in your body.

Pause

You are ready to make small changes in the area of your health... Some of the small changes are eating right... having a control on emotions...and exercising regularly.

And I wonder if you can now paint yourself on a canvas, which is hung on an easel. The painting is of your new slim body, the perfect silhouette, beautiful and attractive.

Paint yourself with a healthier body having a positive vibe and energy.

I am going to stay quiet for a few moments, so that you can paint yourself with the clothes that you would want to wear, looking absolutely gorgeous and confident.

Longer Pause
And, with your imagination...you have the capability to enter into the canvas and enter

the woman you have just drawn and painted.

Imagine yourself on the canvas, looking absolutely gorgeous, confident, hopeful, positive, having a slim and attractive body.

You may want to feel your legs, arms, torso, and chest. See how it feels to be slim. Amazing, isn't it?

With this, you are absolutely sure that to feel amazing, you need to have a slim body. You know that you must change now.

These changes that you are making will have positive effects on your body and life. Imagine what it would be like doing other important things in your life in your new beautiful body.

Feel the confidence you will have once you have achieved the desired body shape and weight. Imagine doing the things you desire to do like adventure sports and other similar such activities that you have always wanted to do but stopped yourself from doing because of the extra weight your carried.

And this how you will live the rest of your life, absolutely confident, positive, with high self-esteem.

I am going to count from 1 to 5 and with each count up, the feelings of confidence, hope, positivity, and self-esteem will double up.

1, 2, 3, 4, and 5.

That's right.

And, say to yourself – " I am slimming" and notice how amazing you feel when you say these words – " I am slimming"

And, every time in future, you want to remind yourself of the journey you are on. Simply say – I am slimming and you will be able to bring back the feelings of confidence, high self-esteem, positivity and hope.

Pause

Anytime, you feel like overeating or skipping the exercise program, say the words I am slimming, and you will be back to the thoughts of losing weight and take the right actions.

Reinforcement Script

And, you continue to drift down...deeper and deeper into...a beautiful comfy feeling...focusing on the sound of my voice and focusing on the goal of achieving your ideal weight.

It is so wonderful to feel relaxed and drift down... into a lovely feeling and as you do so, you can really start to feel good and enjoy this calming space. So perfect to be here and listen to me.

And...you can drop all your tensions and your body knows how to feel relaxed and good and with every breath you take, you find it easier and easier to fall further into this deep relaxation. And your body exactly knows how to feel happy and good and feel relaxed.

Pause

So, just let go and go with the flow and think about nothing, nothing at all as all you need to do is to simply relax and let go...

Pause

And congratulations on your decision to live your life in a healthier way...you have made the decision and commitment to yourself and with the help of hypnosis, we can use the positive reinforcement to help you maintain the motivation to eat healthy and exercise regularly to achieve your ideal goal weight and body.

And because of old habits...you know that you are creating issues for your health and body. And with healthy habits and exercise... you can turn it around and be someone that you always wanted to be. Fit, slimmer, and healthy.

Pause

You overcame all your old limiting beliefs and behaviours and you took charge of your life and this makes you feel great about yourself. Isn't it?

And from today, you look forward a successful future where you see yourself as a positive, healthy, joyful, and confident person. You see yourself as successful.

With every passing day…your old way of living fades away as you continue to move forward through the tunnel and leave behind all that does not serve any purpose and does not belong to you and in front you notice light…the new life awaits. The brighter life, the healthier life is waiting for you.

You are excited and curious to look forward to a successful and healthy life.

And you can achieve the life you desire right now only when you are motivated and determined.

With every passing day, the motivation and determination are getting stronger and stronger.

Pause

You are determined to put healthy nutritious food in your mouth and you chew it at least 10 times. You drink at least 8 glasses of water. You exercise at least 30 minutes every day.

And because you need to take care of your mind, you also need to take care of you mind, to look beautiful inside out. And, that is why you also start to look after your mind. You think happy and remain in the present moment.

Pause

You practice mindfulness and focus on what is at hand instead of thinking about what has gone or what is coming.

Mindfulness or focusing on the here ...and now allows you to be positive and keeps you focused on your weight loss journey. You think positive and feel positive which leads to positive actions.

Pause

You are so happy to have made a decision and commitment to a healthier life. A healthier you await you and in no time, you will be able to meet her soon. The slimmer and happier you. Isn't it?

You are proud of yourself and you deserve to experience the feelings of accomplishment... and with every passing day, you are getting even more determined to meet the everyday goals of eating healthy and exercising regularly.

And as you continue to take actions and see the results, you also inspire people around you. From family and friends, to colleagues and relatives, everyone is surprised to see your determination and they ask you the secrets of losing weight.

Pause

You feel so good already that you are able to accomplish the long-desired goal to lose weight and you can feel the difference in your body and you feel in your old clothes. They are getting lose on you.

Pause

You are excited to change the wardrobe once you reach the ideal goal weight and look your best, aligned to the latest fashion.

Now imagine yourself again at the goal weight you want to be at and see the clothes you are wearing.

Pause

Feel how you are feeling, perhaps liberated, confident, excited, healthier, and happier. Isn't it?

Suggestions/Affirmations

1. You are becoming slimmer and stronger (5 seconds Pause)
2. You are mindful of eating (Same as above)
3. You exercise regularly (Same as above)

4. You sleep well every night and take at least 6 hours of deep sleep (Same as above)
5. You enjoy eating green, dark leafy vegetables (Same as above)
6. Your body is becoming slimmer with every passing day (Same as above)
7. You are in control of your life (Same as above)
8. You have taken charge of your life and body (Same as above)
9. You feel good when you eat healthy and exercise regularly (Same as above)
10. Your body gets rid of extra fat (Same as above)
11. Your love yourself with every passing day (Same as above)
12. You are motivated to achieve your ideal goal weight (Same as above)
13. You avoid high calorie food (Same as above)

14. You enjoy smaller portions of food (Same as above)

15. You chew eat mouthful atleast 10 times and relish the flavors (Same as above)

16. You eat fresh fruits and savor the flavors (Same as above)

17. You look forward to your exercise session every day (Same as above)

18. You are positive (Same as above)

19. You are focused on your daily actions and daily goals (Same as above)

20. You see yourself having the ideal body and weight (Same as above)

21. You stay focused on this weight loss journey (Same as above)

22. You enjoy the taste of fresh fruits (Same as above)

23. You enjoy the taste of veggies (Same as above)

24. You include lean proteins and skimmed milk in your diet (Same as above)

25.You enjoy the taste of salads (Same as above)

26. Your body is becoming slimmer (Same as above)

27. Your stomach and hips are becoming smaller (Same as above)

28.You are getting stronger and leaner (Same as above)

29. You gain muscle and lose weight (Same as above)

30. You feel stronger and stronger with every passing day (Same as above)

31. Your trust your body and it gets easier and easier to trust it (Same as above)

32. Your health is improving with every passing day (Same as above)

33. Making small changes are becoming so much easier for you (Same as above)

34. You are patient and believe in yourself (Same as above)

35. You believe that you will achieve the weight loss goal (Same as above)
36. Letting go of past is easier (Same as above)
37. You are in control of your emotions (Same as above)
38. You are focused and determined (Same as above)
39. You are full of energy (Same as above)
40. You are the creator of your own future (Same as above)
41. You believe your strengths and capabilities (Same as above)
42. You are capable to lose weight (Same as above)
43. You love and accept yourself (Same as above)
44. You are full of self-love (Same as above)
45. You give your body all the nutrients it needs (Same as above)

46. Every day of exercise and eating right food makes you even more confident (Same as above)
47. You are confident (Same as above)
48. You have high self-worth (Same as above)
49. Your love for yourself increases with every passing day (Same as above)
50. You are focused on your weight loss journey (Same as above)

All these suggestions are firmly embedded in your sub-conscious mind and with every passing day, getting stronger and stronger with every passing day, hour, minute.

Waking Up

In a moment, I am going to count you up from one to five and with each count up, you will be back in the present moment and wide awake. Feeling fully refreshed and looking forward to the new you.

Starting now at one, two, three, coming slowly back, four – eyelids beginning to flutter and five – eyes open wide awake.

www.ingramcontent.com/pod-product-compliance
Lightning Source LLC
Chambersburg PA
CBHW071114030426
42336CB00013BA/2079